THE CARDIAC SURGEON'S

Diet & Health Design

01/27/01

JOSH RALEY:

BEST WISHES!

— B P Loughridge

THE CARDIAC SURGEON'S

Diet & Health Design

B.P. LOUGHRIDGE, M.D.
F.A.C.S., F.A.C.C.

CREATIVE SPECIALISTS, INC.

Designer KAREN LITCHFIELD

Project editor LORRI LAGORIN

PRINTED IN THE UNITED STATES OF AMERICA

ISBN 0-9703393-0-5

TO OBTAIN COPIES OF THIS BOOK, PLEASE CALL
TOLL-FREE

1-877-590-DIET

OR ORDER ON THE WORLD WIDE WEB AT
www.dietandhealthdesign.com

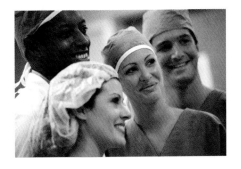

Dedication

This book is dedicated to all the operating room
and intensive care nursing staff with whom I
worked over the years. They made my life and the
lives of my patients infinitely better.

B.P. Loughridge, MD

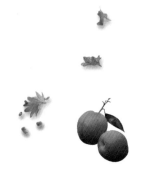

THE CARDIAC SURGEON'S DIET & HEALTH DESIGN

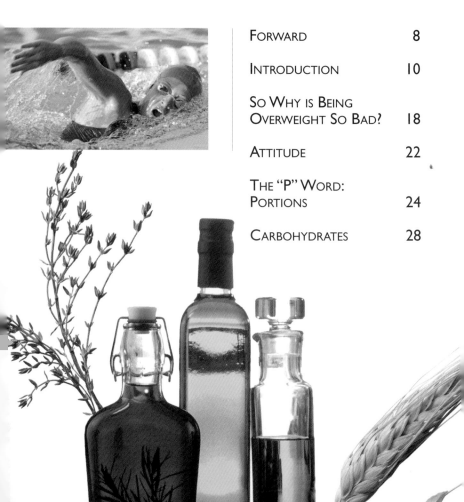

Contents

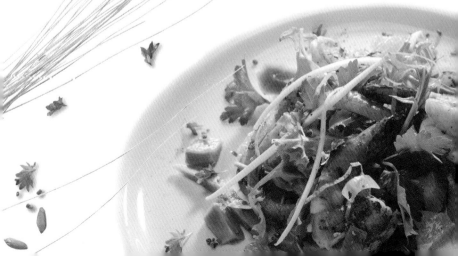

Forward

"MY PEOPLE ARE DESTROYED FOR

LACK OF KNOWLEDGE."

HOSEA 4:6

This little book delivers extremely valuable information and advice to the average American and can help people live better, healthier, and longer lives. Bill P. Loughridge, a cardiovascular surgeon for 28 years, has done remarkable work with outstanding results in his surgical procedures. During his years as a surgeon, Dr. Loughridge has identified different characteristics and clinical entities, as well as risk factors, that contribute to cardiovascular and arteriosclerotic diseases. He has thoroughly reviewed the research and literature in this area and his statements in this book are evidence-based medicine.

As a frequent researcher coming from Europe to the United States, one of the things I have found most striking about

American people is their size. Just looking around when you arrive at the airport, you see an enormous number of men and women who are overweight, and many of them have malignant obesity.

Each individual reading this book can follow the advice about lifestyle changes and thereby decrease in weight or at least not gain weight. Not only is this an enormous benefit for the individual, it also benefits the American health system.

Larsolof Hafsröm
Professor of Surgery
University Hospital
Umeå, Sweden

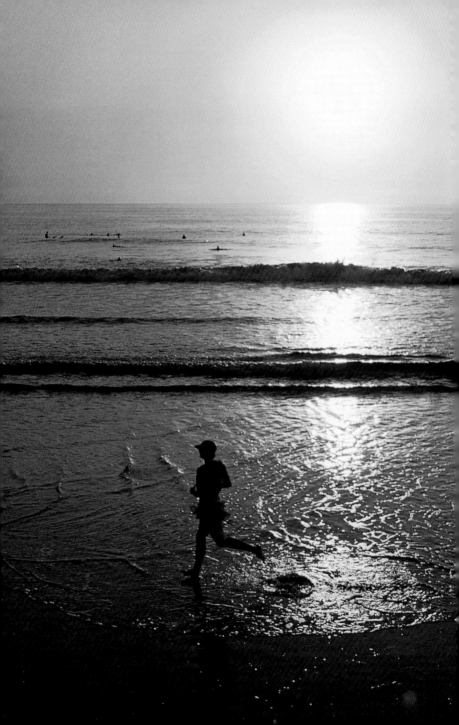

Introduction

Follow the simple plan in this book. You will lose weight, feel better about yourself, have more energy, look better, and have the potential for living a longer, active life— without being hungry.

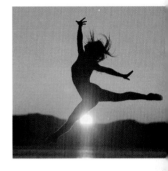

In the early years of my practice as a cardiac surgeon, patients were discharged from the hospital following heart surgery on strict diets of low sodium, minimal fat and meat intake, and high carbohydrates.

At the three-week post-operative evaluation, several findings were clearly evident. Often times, patients were weaker than when they left the hospital. Their blood pressure frequently was too low, and they told of episodes of extreme lethargy and sometimes shakiness about two hours after eating. They also complained that their meals absolutely had very little taste and very little satisfying effect.

As I observed these findings and heard these complaints more and more, I began to investigate certain causative factors, and all evidence pointed to poor nutrition in these post-operative patients.

THE CARDIAC SURGEON'S DIET & HEALTH DESIGN

Consequently, I drastically changed the post-operative dietary regimen for my patients to one very close to what is described in this book. Obviously, this dietary approach was vitamins and mineral supplements, my patients made marked improvements. It became noticeable to other physicians that my patients recovered from surgery much more rapidly

Most farmlands have been overworked, resulting in produce lacking adequate mineral content.

in marked contrast to that prescribed by most physicians.

Once this new dietary program of balanced meals containing protein, carbohydrates, and fat in proper proportion was initiated, along with multi-

than patients who were managed on the low-sodium, low/no fat, high-carbohydrate diet.

Patients on the typical post-operative diet simply were not getting the proper nutrients in the correct proportion. They were, in fact, *undernourished.*

After much study, observation, literature searches, and clinical research regarding nutrition and wellness, it has become obvious to me that this lack of proper

Sounds strange, doesn't it? To be overweight and undernourished. Looking around at shopping malls, airports, movie theaters, or any place where large groups of people congregate, you see

nutrition is a factor in many people's lives, not just those who are recovering from heart surgery.

Wake up, Americans! People are more overweight and under-nourished than they have ever been in this great country.

such an astounding number of obese people: yet these same people are undernourished.

It has become obvious that a marked change is in order for the dietary habits of the American people.

But not all the blame can be placed on our eating habits. As far as nutrition and nourishment go, the majority of the foods we eat are extremely low in certain actual nutritional products, i.e., vitamins and minerals. The beautiful fruits and vegetables we buy are often harvested before any maturation has occurred, hence these products have diminished amounts of vitamins and minerals within them. Also, most of our farmlands are poor in mineral content. Farmers have been aware of the necessity of adding nitrates, phosphates, and potash to the soil for many years. However, most of the farming soil is actually lacking in true mineral content, and thus the fruits and vegetables contain insufficient minerals, which are key elements to maintaining healthy bodily functions and skeletal structure.

As a practicing cardiovascular surgeon for many years, I have had hundreds of discussions with my patients and their families regarding nutrition, diets, lifestyles, and health plans.

It is through the urgings of my patients and their families that I have written this book, which is a compilation of known facts about body weight control and the nutritional requirements necessary to maintain and heal our bodies.

So, how about it? Do you count yourself as one of the *Obese-amoths,* undernourished and overfed? Or do you count yourself as just a "little overweight?" Maybe you're at your ideal weight, and quite healthy.

If you follow the simple plan in this book, you *will* lose weight. You will feel better about yourself, have *more energy, look better*, and have the potential for *living a longer, active life— without being hungry.*

This simple health design
is easy for everyone to
adopt and does not require
food scales for measuring
or calorie counting!

(A Real Life Story)

ONE PATIENT IN PARTICULAR stands out quite clearly in my mind. Dr. E. H., a brilliant and scholarly minister, underwent open heart surgery comprised of prosthetic aortic valve replacement, plus quadruple coronary artery bypass grafting. There was a complicated post-operative course due to a coagulopathy—a blood clotting disorder that sometimes occurs as a result of utilizing the heart lung machine.

During his lengthy stay in the hospital, he became malnourished, eating the standard hospital food of low sodium, very little protein and fat, and a nonflavorful high-carbohydrate diet—of course prepared with no salt and nothing but salt substitute for flavoring.

At his two-week post hospital dismissal appointment, he was extremely weak and shaky with dark circles under his eyes, and his blood pressure was low as compared to his previous blood pressure measurements. After carefully examining him, I could find nothing to account for his extreme weakness and lethargy. I was highly suspicious that Dr. E. H. was indeed in a malnourished state.

He stated that he often became quite lethargic and shaky about two hours following his meal—which was the type of diet prescribed for him in the hospital—low sodium, low protein, almost zero fat, and mainly carbohydrates. He also stated he experienced a "craving" hunger pattern that could not be satisfied with his current diet, and that he "might as well be eating spider legs and butterfly wings."

I asked the laboratory to obtain a blood sample for analysis and invited Dr. E. H. to accompany me on an errand—one that I was sure would change the way he felt.

(A REAL LIFE STORY)

AFTER LEAVING MY OFFICE, WE STOPPED AT A HAMBURGER RESTAURANT. I INVITED DR. E. H. TO COME IN WITH ME. HE LOOKED AT ME AS THOUGH I WAS SOME TYPE OF ALIEN.

WHEN I ORDERED EACH OF US A CHEESEBURGER, DR. E. H. WAS CERTAIN I WAS FROM OUTER SPACE. I HAD TO PRACTICALLY FORCE HIM TO EAT THAT CHEESEBURGER. I EXPLAINED TO HIM THAT THIS WAS NOT TO BE HIS DAILY DIET, BUT THAT THIS WAS A QUICK WAY TO "JUMP-START" HIM TO A POSITIVE NUTRITIONAL STATUS.

WHEN WE FINISHED EATING, I TOOK HIM HOME AND HE INVITED ME IN. WE CHATTED FOR ABOUT AN HOUR, AND HE SUDDENLY EXCLAIMED THAT HE HAD NOT FELT THIS WELL IN MONTHS. I EXPLAINED THAT ENOUGH TIME HAD PASSED FOR SOME OF THE ELEMENTS OF THE CHEESEBURGER TO BE ASSIMILATED BY HIS BODY. I FURTHER DISCUSSED THE PROTEIN, CARBOHYDRATES, AND FAT BALANCED MEAL PROGRAM WITH HIS WIFE AND HIM, WHO SUBSEQUENTLY IMPLEMENTED THE MEAL DESIGN. THIS NEW DIET PROVIDED A MOST RAPID AND SATISFACTORY OVERALL RECOVERY. TO THIS DAY, DR. E. H. FOLLOWS THE DIETARY DESIGN THAT I OUTLINED FOR HIM 20 YEARS AGO.

So Why is Being Overweight So Bad?

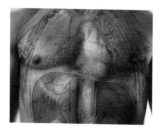

Many people who are overweight say, "Why should I lose weight? I'm happy the way I am."

While, in theory it may be true—you can be overweight and still be happy—the reality of the situation is by being significantly overweight or obese you are increasing the likelihood of developing many serious, sometimes fatal illnesses.

Several disease entities are related to the overweight/obese health categories, including:

- High blood pressure
- Diabetes
- Gallbladder disease
- Osteoarthritis
- Heart Disease
- Certain types of cancer

In an interesting analysis of Body Mass Index related to mortality, Stevens et al reported that moderate obesity may generally result in a one—to

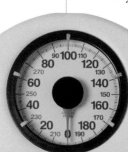

HOW MUCH WEIGHT IS OVERWEIGHT?

THE WORLD HEALTH ORGANIZATION AND NATIONAL INSTITUTES OF HEALTH, AS WELL AS MOST SKILLED NUTRITIONISTS AND NUTRITIONAL INVESTIGATORS, USE THE BODY MASS INDEX (BMI) AS THE FRAME OF REFERENCE FOR PROPER BODY WEIGHT ASSESSMENTS. BMI IS CALCULATED AS WEIGHT IN KGS (1 KG = 2.205 LBS OR 1 LB = .4535 KG) DIVIDED BY THE SQUARE OF HEIGHT IN METERS (1 INCH = 2.54 CM AND 100 CM = 1 METER). FOR EXAMPLE, THE BMI FOR A 5'8" MALE WEIGHING 155 LBS IS AS FOLLOWS:

5'8" = 68 INCHES
68 INCHES (2.54 CM/IN) = 172.72 CM OR 1.73 METERS ROUNDED
1.73^2 = 2.9929 CM OR 3 METERS ROUNDED
155 LBS (.45/LB) = 69.75KG OR 70 KG ROUNDED
70 KG (WEIGHT) DIVIDED BY 3 M (HEIGHT) = 23.33
THUS CALCULATED **BMI is 23.33**

- **BMI of < 20** = VERY LOW AMOUNT OF BODY FAT, SEEN IN WELL CONDITIONED ATHLETES OR SERIOUSLY ILL, CACHECTIC INDIVIDUALS.
- **BMI of 20 - 22** = IDEAL, HEALTHY AMOUNT OF FAT -- AESTHETICALLY ATTRACTIVE, LOWEST INCIDENCE OF FAT RELATED ILLNESSES.
- **BMI of 22 - 25** = ACCEPTABLE RANGE, BUT BORDERLINE.
- **BMI of 25 - 30** = OVERWEIGHT, SOME INVESTIGATORS CALL THIS CATEGORY OBESE. THERE IS AN ASSOCIATED RISK OF INCREASED EARLY MORTALITY AND AN INCREASED INCIDENCE OF CERTAIN ILLNESSES.
- **BMI > 30** = MORBIDLY OBESE, INCREASED RISK FOR DIABETES, HIGH BLOOD PRESSURE, GALLBLADDER DISEASE, HEART DISEASE, OSTEOARTHRITIS, AND CERTAIN CANCERS.

BASED ON THE THIRD NATIONAL HEALTH AND NUTRITION EXAMINATION SURVEY (NHANES III) DATA, APPROXIMATELY 63% OF MEN AND 55% OF WOMEN AGED 25 YEARS OR OLDER IN THE UNITED STATES ARE OVERWEIGHT OR OBESE. FURTHERMORE, THE PERCENTAGE OF OBESE PEOPLE IN THE UNITED STATES HAS INCREASED FROM 14.5 PERCENT IN THE YEARS 1976-1980, TO 22.5 PERCENT IN 1988-1994, TO 50 PERCENT IN 1999.

ACCORDING TO THIS STUDY, THE EPIDEMIC OF OBESITY IN THE UNITED STATES RESULTS FROM SOCIETAL DIETARY HABITS AND LIFESTYLE.

three-year *reduction of life expectancy,* depending upon age.

High Blood Cholesterol levels are very prevalent in people who fall into the overweight or obese

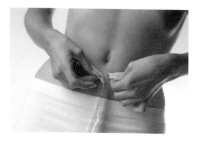

categories. This is probably related to the high-carbohydrate meals generally ingested by overweight/obese individuals.

There is no question that obesity is a major cause of mortality in the United States, and in addition to the mortality rate, overweight-obesity certainly significantly increases *morbidity* and definitely *impairs your quality of life.*

A study by Ming Wei, et al., indicates that when compared to

men of normal weight, obese men have an almost three-fold higher risk of a cardiovascular event.

Some people may be overweight as a result of a congenital hormone imbalance in which they lack the hormone *leptin.* The protein hormone leptin is important to the homeostatic regulation of body fat and individuals who have a genetic deficiency of leptin do exhibit extreme obesity. However, this condition is extremely rare, and in most cases, is *not* likely the cause of obesity.

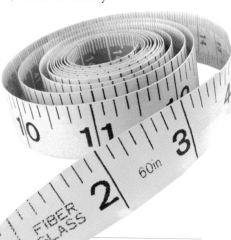

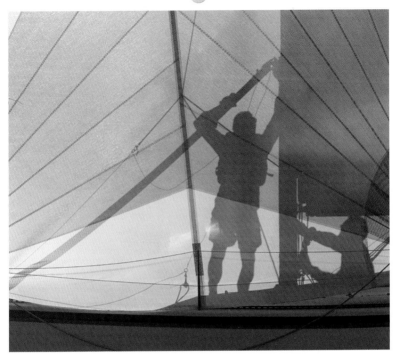

The good news is you can take steps now to regain your health and get back on track to a healthy lifestyle. The health design outlined in this book offers a remedy for this epidemic of pandemic proportions; so implement this design, and you will experience the exhilaration of wellness, ideal body weight, and opportunity for increased longevity. Remember, you are responsible for you.

So, what do you say?

Do it for your family, do it for your spouse, do it for yourself— what ever it takes. Just do it, and see what a difference it will make in your life.

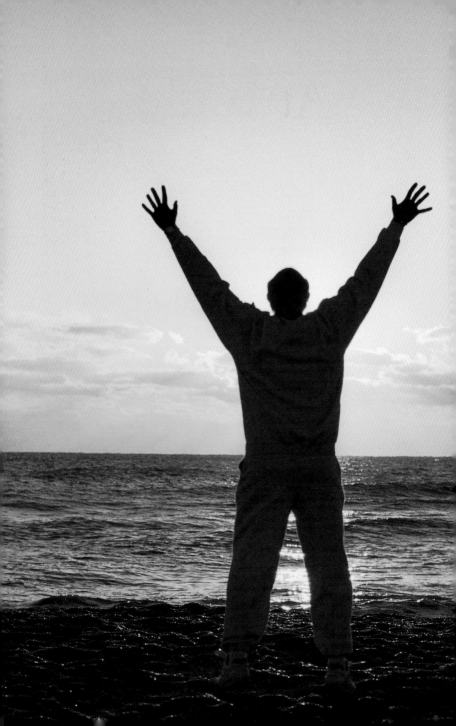

Attitude

"I am responsible for changing the things in my health and appearance that can be changed."

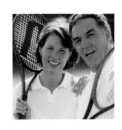

The first step and principal component to a healthy body is a commitment to being *accountable* for your own nutrition and lifestyle.

Establish the attitude that *"I am responsible* for changing the things in my health and appearance that can be changed. I am responsible for the quantities and types of food that I ingest. I am responsible for learning about protein, carbohydrates, fat, and vitamin and mineral requirements, as well as exercise—all of which are necessary to develop and maintain a healthy body."

This attitude requires a lifelong commitment that can easily be accomplished without being radical or fanatical in your approach to a healthy lifestyle. Also, this new attitude allows you to not only be healthier, but to be happier with an improvement in appearance and self-esteem.

Bear in mind that moderation and balance in your approach to health allows you to *sustain* your healthy program, thus preventing a "burn-out" and a return to your old lifestyle.

Now, let's move forward with this new attitude and commitment to accountability!

Portions,

America has
always been known
as the "land of
plenty," but today as
Americans stretch
and strain the seams
of their pants, this
reputation for over
indulgence is catching up
to us.

We have become a nation
ruled by instant gratification
when it comes to food, as

The "P" Word – Portions, Portions!

One of the most important factors in being overweight is the consumption of large portions of food.

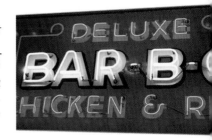

evidenced by the plethora of fast food restaurants. Coupled with this rapid serving of our meals are enormous quantities of food. We feel we must "get our money's worth," so we expect large portions of food, and certainly, since we paid for this meal, we feel we should eat it all —*wrong!*

The most important factor in being overweight is the consumption of large portions of

food. In addition, eating improper ratios of protein, carbohydrates, and fat also contributes to America's weighty problem, which will be discussed later.

The average person should consume between 1500 and 2500 calories per day—depending on their level of physical activity and body size. Obviously, those individuals who lead sedentary lifestyles require fewer calories, but often times, these individuals are the ones who are most overweight. To put that number of calories in perspective, a typical fast food specialty burger—two beef patties, various sauces, lettuce, pickles, ketchup, mustard, and the works, topped off by a bun—can tip the calorie scale at over 1,000 calories all by itself. Add to that the "bigger is better" size French fries, and you have well over the amount of calories you need for the entire day.

Bear in mind that this caloric load is primarily in the form of carbohydrates, which is a major factor in the obesity problem of Americans that will be addressed later in the book.

So, what are the proper portions and proportions necessary to avoid over eating? And how can you implement them without carrying a measuring cup and scale with you at all times?

It's simple. A "Rule of Thumb" or better yet, a *Rule of Hand"* is to eat a meal no larger than your hand.

Simply observe the palm of your hand as well as its thickness. This will be your guideline for your meal portion. This measurement will closely determine your

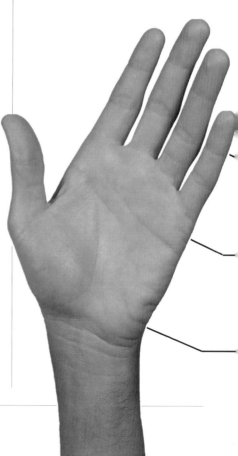

optimal portion and proportion requirement of protein, carbohydrates, and fats at each meal for it will correlate with each individual's size.

Next, visually divide your hand into one-thirds and allocate 1/3 volume to protein, 1/3 volume to carbohydrates, and

1/3 volume to fat containing food.

Remember, proper diet balance and portion is not an exact science and it does not require exact calorie counting and measurements. You don't need to count calories or guess at how big a portion constitutes three or four ounces.

However, the system does require you have knowledge of which foods are protein, carbohydrates, and fat. This will be addressed for you later in this book.

Read the labels on food products and use the "Rule of Hand." You will lose excess weight, develop more energy, and experience an improved self-image with a sensation of overall wellness.

Now, let's explore the three macronutrients of our diets—protein, carbohydrates, and fat.

1/3 PROTEIN

1/3 CARBOHYDRATES

1/3 FAT CONTAINING FOOD

Carbohydrates

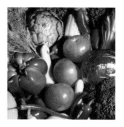

Americans have been so indoctrinated to eliminate fatty foods from their daily diets, they have gone overboard on the consumption of carbohydrates.

Unfortunately, this over-indulgence of carbohydrates has resulted in a nation of over-weight, obese individuals who are actually poorly nourished.

To understand the role carbo-hydrates have played in the American diet, it is important to understand the role carbo-hydrates play in your body. Carbohydrates are basically sugars that are broken down into glucose, which is stored first as glycogen

CARBOHYDRATES: WHAT ARE THEY?
They are sugar compounds made by plants!

SUGARS	**STARCHES**	**FIBERS**
SIMPLE CARBOHYDRATES	COMPLEX CARBOHYDRATES	CELLULOSE & PECTIN
Sugars are termed **simple** *carbohydrates. Examples — refined sugar, milk products, honey, natural fruit sugars.*	*Starches are called* **complex** *carbohydrates. Examples — grains, fruits, potatoes, and other vegetables.*	*Fiber is essentially not digested thus it provides no caloric contribution. Examples — fruits, vegetables, legumes, grains.*
TABLE SUGAR	BREAD	BRAN
HONEY	CEREALS	POPCORN
VEGETABLE	CRACKERS	BREADS
MILK	FLOUR	CORN
ICE CREAM	LEGUMES (BEANS)	OATS
CARBONATED BEVERAGES	RICE	RICE
CANDY	POTATOES	BEANS
FRUITS — FRESH & DRIED	PASTA	NUTS
PUDDINGS	PIE CRUSTS	LETTUCE
PIES	NUTS	CELERY
		APPLES
		BERRIES
		PEARS
		STRAWBERRIES
		PLUMS
		APRICOTS
		PEAS
		POTATOES
		BROCCOLI
		SQUASH

DIETARY FIBER

Dietary fiber reduces insulin secretion by slowing the rate of nutrient absorption following a meal. Dietary fiber exerts a major effect on the glycemic, and therefore, the insulinemic (amount of insulin in the bloodstream) response to carbohydrates in a meal.

in the liver and muscles. After the storage areas in the liver and muscle are full of glycogen, any excess carbohydrate stimulates *insulin,* which is basically a *storage hormone* and the excess carbohydrate is then *stored as body fat.*

Body fat is not utilized until the glycogen stores in the liver are diminished with resulting low blood sugars, which trigger a release of glucagon hormone from the pancreas. Glucagon is the antithesis of insulin and thus mobilizes stored body fat for metabolism into glucose and thus energy.

Since glucagon offsets the action of insulin, it is the dominant amount of these hormones in the bloodstream that determines whether or not you gain or lose excess body fat.

TWO TYPES OF DIETARY FIBER

SOLUBLE

Beta-glucans in oats and barley and pectin in apples—there is some evidence indicating these fibers help lower cholesterol.

INSOLUBLE

Cellulose and lignin found in whole grains—acts as natural laxative.

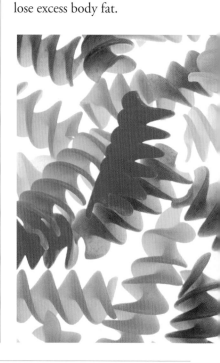

The amount of stored body fat is based upon the amount of insulin released into the bloodstream and the amount of insulin released is based upon the amount of incoming carbohydrates.

In essence, increased amounts of incoming carbohydrates result in increased amounts of insulin, which in turn takes the carbohydrate load and stores it as body fat. Further, as you continue to load your diet with breads, pastas, cereals, etc., the resulting increased amounts of insulin secreted *prevent* the already *stored* body fat from being metabolized and used as energy, thus compounding the obesity problem.

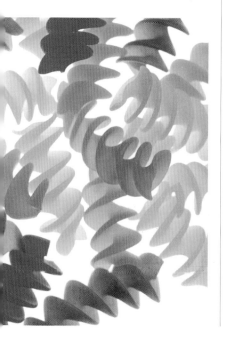

Breads, pastas, potatoes, cereals, etc. are carbohydrates which are *rapidly* broken down and converted to glucose, which in turn causes increased amounts of insulin to be secreted and thus increasing stored body fat. These carbohydrates are not to be avoided, but should be eaten in *moderation.*

It is noteworthy that carbohydrates are necessary for proper brain function, but on the other hand, carbohydrate overload releases too much insulin, which then drives down the blood sugar below a level where one's brain functions effectively. This is why even though we may feel an initial charge of energy, or "sugar high," we become lethargic and sleepy after a large carbohydrate-loaded meal.

You must also remember that fruits and vegetables are also carbohydrates but these are preferred types since they are comprised mainly of fructose which first must be converted by the liver before absorption can occur as glucose. This is a much slower process and results in slower and lower insulin release, thus resulting in less stored body fat.

Even if you eat only fruits and vegetables as the primary source of carbohydrates, you must be cognizant of *portions* eaten to prevent carbohydrate overload.

All you really need to remember is this: carbohydrate overload results in too much stored body fat. Also, you should try to use fruits and vegetables as your main sources of carbohydrates because they trigger a slightly slower release of insulin than some of the other carbohydrates.

Excess Carbohydrates
↓
Excess Insulin
↓
Excess Storage of Body Fat

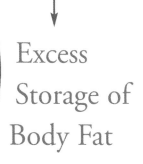

ACTION OF INSULIN	ACTION OF GLUCAGON
Decreases elevated blood sugar	Increases low blood sugar
Triggers the body's metabolism into storage action	Triggers body's metabolism into utilization of stored products
Changes glucose and protein to stored fat	Changes fat and protein into glucose
Changes dietary fat to stored fat	Changes dietary fat to ketones for tissue energy
Raises body's production of cholesterol	Lowers the body's production of cholesterol

33

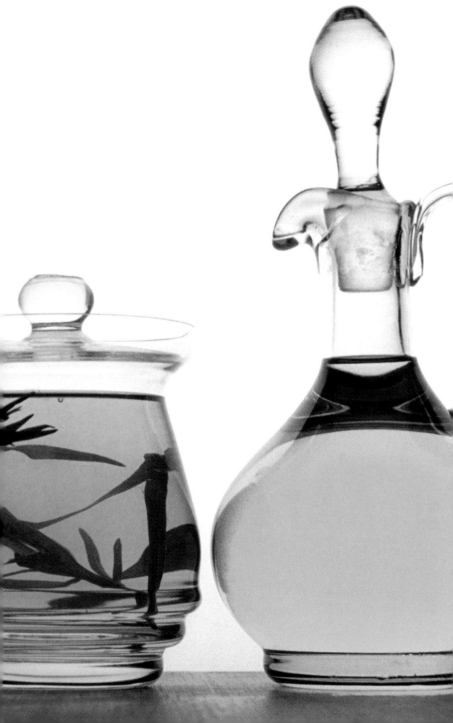

Fat

Dietary fat in moderation is a natural and desirable part of a healthy eating design.

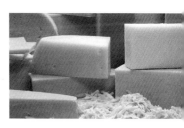

Fat has become the proverbial "Bad Word" of the 1990s, with everyone from preteens to senior citizens trying to eliminate fat from their diets. However, including fat in meals not only adds to the flavor of your meal, but also is very beneficial in diminishing your stored body fat.

It seems paradoxical doesn't it? But fat is hormonally important in achieving dietary balance.

Fat slows the absorption and entry pathways of glucose into the bloodstream. This, in turn, slows the secretion of insulin, which slows the deposition of stored body fat, actually enhanc-ing the use of the already stored body fat. Here's how it works.

When fat reaches your small intestine, a hormone named *cholecystokinin* is released. This hormone tells the hunger center in your brain that you have eaten enough food, thus suppressing your appetite. Cholecystokinin also signals the release of bile salts and lipase, which help breakdown fats into fatty acids and glycerol and further depress the appetite. Eating slowly and waiting a few seconds after each bite allows this impor-tant hormonal pathway to curb your appetite.

DIETARY FATS

THE FOOD FATS ARE MADE UP OF A COMBINATION OF FATTY ACIDS. A FOOD FAT IS LABELED AS "SATURATED," "MONOUNSATURATED," OR "POLYUNSATURATED." YOU HAVE NO DOUBT HEARD OF ALL OF THESE TYPES OF FAT, BUT DO YOU KNOW WHAT TYPES OF FOOD CONTAIN DIFFERENT KINDS OF FAT? DO YOU KNOW WHICH TYPE OF FATS YOU NEED TO AVOID AND WHICH ARE MORE ACCEPTABLE IN YOUR DIET? A FOOD FAT IS LABELED ACCORDING TO THE CHEMICAL STRUCTURE OF THE FATTY ACIDS IT CONTAINS AND THE ATTACHMENT OF THE HYDROGEN ATOMS TO THE FAT MOLECULE.

- When the chemical bonds of the fat have a hydrogen atom attached to ALL of the carbon atoms, the fat is said to be SATURATED.
- When the bonds can hold additional hydrogen atoms, the fat is UNSATURATED.
- A MONOUNSATURATED fat forms one double bond between two carbon atoms.
- A POLYUNSATURATED fatty acid forms several double bonds between several carbon atoms by dropping off hydrogen atoms and allowing a single hydrogen atom to attach to more than one carbon atom.

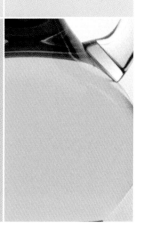

For those of you with *fat phobia*—those who live by the no-fat rule, eating mainly carbohydrates and avoiding fat in the diet in an attempt to decrease the amount of cholesterol concentration in the blood—here is an interesting fact to be considered.

It has been shown by many reliable clinical studies beginning as far back as 1964, where it was reported by Milton Winitz and his associates, that the ingestion of sucrose (carbohydrate) clearly leads to an increase in the cholesterol concentration in the blood.

SATURATED FATS	SATURATED FATS ARE SOLID AT ROOM TEMPERATURE AND GET FIRMER WHEN THEY ARE CHILLED. AN EXAMPLE OF SATURATED FATS IS BUTTER. DIETS HIGH IN SATURATED FATS INCREASE THE AMOUNT OF CHOLESTEROL IN YOUR BLOOD, WHICH HAS BEEN SHOWN TO INCREASE THE RISK OF HEART DISEASE AND STROKE.
MONOUNSATURATED FATS	MONOUNSATURATED FATS ARE LIQUID AT ROOM TEMPERATURE AND THEY THICKEN WHEN CHILLED. AN EXAMPLE OF MONOUNSATURATED FATS IS OLIVE OIL. A DIET HIGH IN UNSATURATED FATS REDUCES THE AMOUNT OF SERUM CHOLESTEROL IN YOUR BLOOD, THUS REDUCING THE RISK OF HEART DISEASE AND STROKE IN COMPARISON TO SATURATED FATS.
POLYUNSATURATED FATS	POLYUNSATURATED FATS ARE LIQUID AT ROOM TEMPERATURE AND STAY LIQUID WHEN THEY ARE CHILLED. AN EXAMPLE OF A POLYUNSATURATED FAT IS CORN OIL. A DIET HIGH IN THIS TYPE OF FAT ALSO LOWERS YOUR RISK OF HEART DISEASE AND STROKE IN COMPARISON TO THE SATURATED FATS.

In another study, John C. Yudkin and his co-workers in a large-scale, long-term epidemiological study of the population of Framingham, Massachusetts, found that people who developed coronary disease had been ingesting more ordinary sugar —a carbohydrate—than those who had not developed the disease. The individuals who had not developed coronary disease ate "balanced" meals, which frequently contained fatty foods. This sucrose/cholesterol effect has its biochemical basis in the fact that certain reactions occur during the metabolic processing

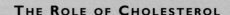

THE ROLE OF CHOLESTEROL

IT IS IMPORTANT TO UNDERSTAND WHAT CHOLESTEROL IS AND HOW IT IS TRANSFERRED THROUGH YOUR SYSTEM. ELEVATED CHOLESTEROL LEVELS HAVE UNEQUIVOCALLY BEEN LINKED TO HEART DISEASE, STROKE, AND PERIPHERAL VASCULAR DISEASE. CHOLESTEROL IS TRANSFERRED THROUGHOUT YOUR BODY IN LIPOPROTEINS, WHICH ARE A COMBINATION OF FAT AND PROTEIN PARTICLES. THERE ARE FOUR TYPES OF LIPOPROTEINS:

- CHYLOMICRONS—VERY LITTLE PROTEIN, LOTS OF FATS
- LOW-DENSITY LIPOPROTEIN, OR LDL—SLIGHTLY MORE PROTEIN THAN CHYLOMICRONS, AND HIGH FAT LEVELS
- VERY LOW-DENSITY LIPOPROTEIN, OR VLDL—MINISCULE PROTEIN AND LARGE AMOUNTS OF FAT
- HIGH DENSITY LIPOPROTEIN, OR HDL—PROPORTIONALLY MORE PROTEIN THAN FAT

THE VERY LOW-DENSITY LIPOPROTEINS (VLDL) AND LOW-DENSITY LIPOPROTEINS (LDL) CARRY CHOLESTEROL THROUGH THE WALLS OF YOUR ARTERIES WHERE IT IS SOMETIMES DEPOSITED. THIS DEPOSIT BUILDS UP AND MAY EVENTUALLY OBSTRUCT THE BLOOD FLOW THROUGH THE ARTERY, RESULTING IN HEART ATTACK, STROKE, OR POOR BLOOD SUPPLY TO OTHER AREAS OF THE BODY.

A DIET HIGH IN SATURATED FATS INCREASES THE AMOUNT OF CHOLESTEROL AND LOW-DENSITY LIPOPROTEINS IN YOUR BLOODSTREAM, AND THIS IS HARMFUL TO YOUR HEALTH AND WELL-BEING.

THE HIGH-DENSITY LIPOPROTEINS (HDL) HAVE BEEN SHOWN TO HELP REMOVE CHOLESTEROL DEPOSITS FROM ARTERIAL WALLS. SO, IT IS IMPORTANT TO HAVE HIGH LEVELS OF HDL IN YOUR BLOODSTREAM. ONE WAY OF RAISING THIS HDL LEVEL IS EXERCISING. EXERCISING ON A REGULAR BASIS ELEVATES THE SERUM LEVEL OF HDL—THAT IN ITSELF SHOULD BE ENOUGH TO GET YOU INTO AN EXERCISE PROGRAM!

of sucrose, whereby some of the products are converted to *cholesterol.*

So, you need to keep away from the sugar bowl, eat those carbohydrate sucrose foods *sparingly,* and always employ the "Rule of Hand"—protein, carbohydrates, and fat in proper proportions—1/3, 1/3, 1/3.

Once again, you are trying to achieve a balance in your diet, which is physiologically sound. To do this, some fat is necessary in your diet. Now, that doesn't mean you need to rush out and order that double cheeseburger and fries just to keep your fat intake up. It simply means that allowing some dietary fat is a

---

TWO IMPORTANT POLYUNSATURATED FATTY ACIDS

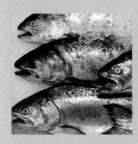

1. OMEGA-6 (LINOLEIC ACID)—OMEGA-6 IS USED IN MAKING PROSTAGLANDINS, WHICH ARE HORMONE-LIKE SUBSTANCES THAT REGULATE MANY ACTIVITIES IN THE BODY INCLUDING KIDNEY FUNCTION, INFLAMMATORY RESPONSES, AND BLOOD CLOTTING MECHANISMS. GOOD SOURCES OF OMEGA-6 ARE PLANTS AND FISH.

2. OMEGA-3 (LINOLENIC ACID)—OMEGA-3 IS IMPORTANT IN LOWERING TRIGLYCERIDE AND CHOLESTEROL LEVELS, LOWERING BLOOD PRESSURE, AND PREVENTING BLOOD CLOTS. GOOD SOURCES OF OMEGA-3 ARE NUTS, SOYBEANS, CANOLA OIL, FLAXSEED OIL, AND COLD WATER FISH.

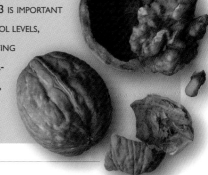

natural and desirable part of a healthy eating design.

It is highly recommended, however, to keep saturated fats—the fatty foods that significantly contribute to buildup of plaque in your arteries—at a minimum in your diet. You need to avoid consuming *large* amounts of fatty red meat, egg yolks, and various organ meats that are high in arachidonic acid, which is harmful to your cardiovascular system.

So remember, in order to achieve dietary balance, some fat is beneficial, but only in moderation.

BEST DIETARY FATS

THE FOLLOWING ARE EXAMPLES OF MONOUNSATURATED FATS, WHICH ARE THE BEST CHOICES OF DIETARY FATS.

Olive oil

Fish oil

Macadamia nut oil

Flaxseed oil

Canola oil

Walnut oil

Avocado oil

Grapeseed oil

THESE EXAMPLES OFFER AN EXTRA BENEFIT OF CONTAINING ANTI-OXIDANTS THAT HELP PROTECT YOUR ARTERIES.

FISH OIL AND CANOLA OIL ARE RICH IN OMEGA-3 FATTY ACIDS, WHICH DECREASE PLATELET AGGREGATION AND BLOOD CLOT FORMATION.

POLYUNSATURATED FATS ARE SECOND CHOICES FOR DIETARY FATS. PROBLEMS WITH POLYUNSATURATED FATS ARISE WHEN THESE FATS ARE HYDROGENATED, SUCH AS THE CASE IN MARGARINE, THEY ACT THE SAME AS THE HARMFUL SATURATED FATS AND MAY RAISE CHOLESTEROL LEVELS.

Protein

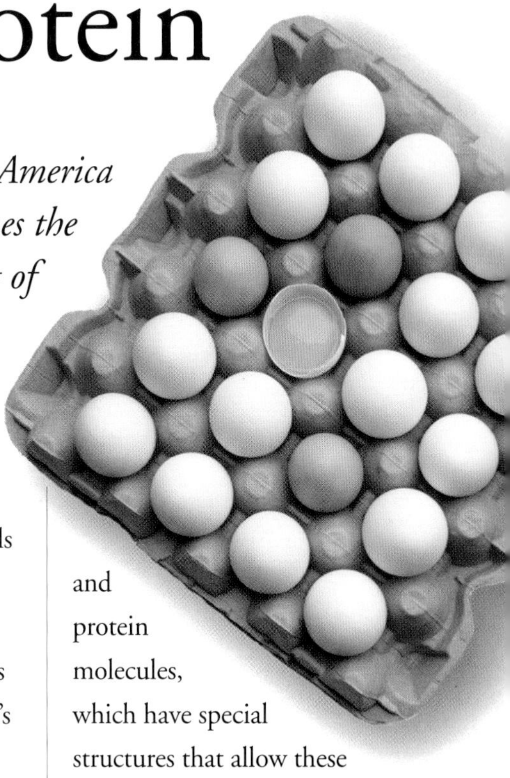

*Most adults in America
eat two to three times the
recommended amount of
protein.*

Among the most important substances in plants and animals are proteins which, when ingested, are broken down into amino acids. These amino acids are building blocks of the body's tissues, and they join together with other substances to make up your structural framework such as hair, fingernails, skin, tendon, muscle, and collagen, which acts to hold everything together.

Blood contains many hundreds of varieties of proteins and protein molecules, which have special structures that allow these proteins to carry out specific and finite tasks. Proteins are eaten, then broken down by our digestive system into amino acids, then, assimilated by our bodies back into proteins.

Certain amino acids that *must* be obtained from your food are called essential amino acids; these are histidine, leucine, isoleucine, lysine, methionine, phenylalamine, threonine, valine, and tryptophan. These essential amino acids are found in meat, fish, and eggs, which should be eaten as a *varied diet* since certain foods are higher in certain essential amino acids than others.

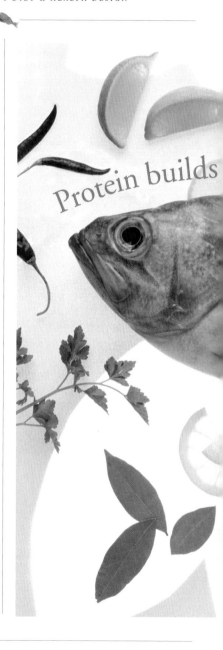

Protein builds

PROTEIN QUALITY

A **COMPLETE PROTEIN** IS ONE THAT CONTAINS ADEQUATE AMOUNTS OF AMINO ACIDS ESSENTIAL TO HUMAN HEALTH. FOOD FROM ANIMALS AND SOYBEANS SUPPLY COMPLETE PROTEINS.

AN **INCOMPLETE PROTEIN** DOES NOT CONTAIN ADEQUATE AMOUNTS OF ESSENTIAL AMINO ACIDS TO SUSTAIN HUMAN WELLNESS. PROTEINS FROM FRUITS, GRAINS, AND VEGETABLES ARE INCOMPLETE WITH THE EXCEPTION OF SOYBEANS WHICH CONTAIN COMPLETE PROTEINS.

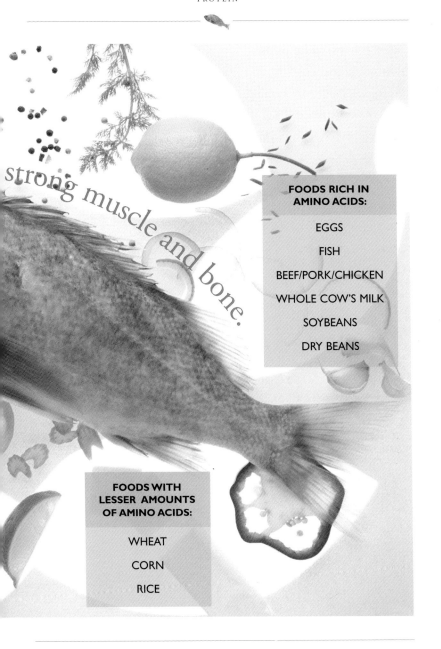

strong muscle and bone.

**FOODS RICH IN
AMINO ACIDS:**

EGGS

FISH

BEEF/PORK/CHICKEN

WHOLE COW'S MILK

SOYBEANS

DRY BEANS

**FOODS WITH
LESSER AMOUNTS
OF AMINO ACIDS:**

WHEAT

CORN

RICE

Ironically, another much maligned food—the egg—has been arbitrarily established by nutritional scientists as the "Protein Gold Standard" against which all other protein containing foods are measured by since other foods generally lack adequate amounts of one or more amino acids.

It is important to note that all proteins are nitrogenous substances, which means that when proteins are broken down in the body, one of these resultant products is urea, which must be excreted through the kidneys. A large dietary intake of protein means a large amount of urea must be excreted by the kidneys. This continued and protracted high blood level of urea *may be harmful to the kidneys*. So, once again, moderation must be applied to your dietary habits.

Most adults in America eat two to

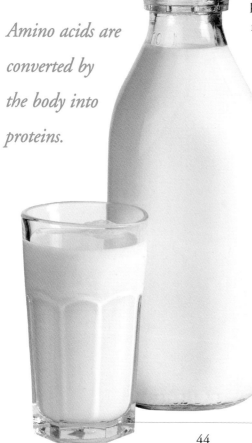

Amino acids are converted by the body into proteins.

three times the recommended amount of protein, and this excess causes no harm provided the kidneys are healthy and provided there are ample amounts of vitamin B12, vitamin B6, and folic acid on board (see chapter on Homocysteine). The excess protein is simply burned as energy along with the fats and carbohydrates or is stored as additional body fat.

You must remain mindful of the proper portions and proportions of protein, carbohydrates, and fat to keep from being or becoming overweight.

If you indulge in unusual or extreme amounts of exercise, if you are a diabetic, or if you desire an interim snack during the day, the same ratio of the snack foods must be 1/3 protein, 1/3 carbohydrates and 1/3 fat. This ratio prevents the glucose/ insulin roller coaster response as previously discussed.

THE TWO TYPES OF AMINO ACIDS

ESSENTIAL
THE BODY CANNOT SYNTHESIZE THESE AND THEY MUST BE OBTAINED FROM FOOD.

NON-ESSENTIAL
THESE AMINO ACIDS CAN BE MANUFACTURED BY THE BODY FROM FATS, CARBOHYDRATES, AND OTHER AMINO ACIDS.

ESSENTIAL AMINO ACIDS:
Must be obtained from food

HISTADINE	PHENYLALANINE
LEUCINE	THREONINE
ISOLEUCINE	TRYPTOPHAN
LYSINE	VALINE
METHIONINE	

NON-ESSENTIAL AMINO ACIDS:
Can be assimilated by the body

ALANINE	ARGININE
ASPARTIC ACID	HYDROXYPROLINE
NORLEUCINE	CITRULLINE
PROLINE	CYSTINE
SERINE	GLUTAMIC ACID
TYROSINE	GLYCINE
HYDROXYGLUTAMIC ACID	

Menu

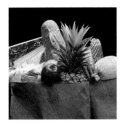

Keep it flexible, but remember portions, and the proper ratio of protein, carbohydrates, and fat.

Visualize the "Rule of Hand" when planning meals, and note that a balanced meal does not require exact measurements.

If you prepare more protein food than you need to eat, use it in the next day's meal plan.

If you think this is not enough food, then you probably *eat too much!*

If you feel you need a mid-day snack, be certain it is in the proper ratio: 1/3 Protein, 1/3 Carbohydrate, 1/3 Fat and *remember, small portions for snacks!*

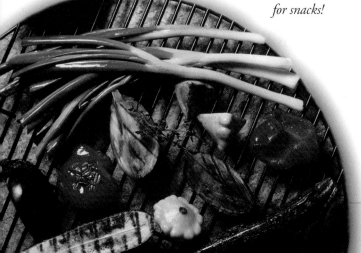

SCRAMBLED EGGS AND BACON

PROTEIN   2 to 6 Egg Whites *(Depending on the size of your hand)*
                   Or 1/2 - 3/4 cup of Egg Substitute
                   2 Slices of Bacon

CARBOHYDRATE   1/2 Slice of Buttered Toast
                   1/4 Cantaloupe

FAT   1 Tsp Olive Oil – Used For Cooking Eggs
                   Bacon Slices *(Above)*

GRILLED CHICKEN SALAD

PROTEIN   4 ounces Shredded Grilled Chicken *(Visualize hand ratio)*
CARBOHYDRATE   Shredded Lettuce
                   Tomatoes
                   Croutons or 1/2 Slice of Bread
FAT   4 Tsp Vinegar and Olive Oil Dressing
                   A Dusting of Parmesan Cheese

PORK MEDALLIONS

PROTEIN   Approximately 4 ounces Pork Loin – Grilled or Baked
                   (Visualize hand size and 1/3 portion size)
CARBOHYDRATE   1/2 cup of Apple Sauce
                   Approximately 1 – 1/2 cup Green Beans
                   (Depending upon hand size)
                   Shredded Lettuce, Tomatoes, and Celery
FAT   4 Tsp Vinegar and Olive Oil Dressing for Salad

Vitamins = Life

*How much of each
vitamin do we
really need?*

Ah,
yes, vitamins.
So named because with-
out these special substances, we
are unable to sustain life.

Interestingly, many people are
not aware that the RDA (required daily allowance) for
vitamins was established as a
guideline to tell us that it is
necessary to ingest vitamins on a
daily basis at the RDA level to
prevent us from becoming ill.
That is not to say that the

established RDA for vitamins is
adequate in amounts to *keep* you
healthy and make you as healthy
as you might be. For example, for
many years the RDA for vitamin
C was 60 mg/day. Only recently
did the American Medical Association recommend increasing
the RDA to 100 mg/day.

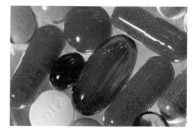

So, how much of each vitamin do we really need? And what's the best way to get those vitamins?

For many years physicians were reluctant to recommend vitamin supplements at all because it was felt that individuals on balanced diets obtained all the vitamins necessary to reach the RDA levels. It has only been recently shown that increased levels of certain vitamins are very beneficial to our cardiovascular system.

Unfortunately, our food sources today are very low in vitamin content. Most of our fruits and vegetables have been harvested prior to maturation and thus the products we eat are low in vitamins. In addition, most Americans don't eat the recommended amounts of vitamin-rich fruits and vegetables they need to stay healthy.

THE NEED FOR VITAMIN SUPPLEMENTS

THE LAST SEVERAL YEARS HAVE SEEN A MARKED INCREASE IN THE NUMBER OF REPRODUCIBLE AND VERIFIABLE SCIENTIFIC STUDIES OF THE RELATIONSHIP AMONG CERTAIN VITAMINS, MINERALS, AND DISEASE PREVENTION.

THE SECOND NATIONAL HEALTH AND NUTRITION EXAMINATION SURVEY (NHANES II) RECENTLY DEMONSTRATED SEVERAL FINDINGS.

FOR EXAMPLE:

1. MANY AMERICANS DIETS DO NOT MEET THE RDA FOR VITAMIN E WHICH IS AN IMPORTANT ANTIOXIDANT. NEARLY 50% OF THE POPULATION HAVE A DAILY INTAKE OF VITAMIN E THAT IS LESS THAN 70% OF THE RDA.

2. ON THE AVERAGE, AT LEAST 72% OF THE ADULT POPULATION DO NOT INGEST FRUITS OR VEGETABLES THAT ARE HIGH IN VITAMIN C AND 80% OF THE ADULTS DO NOT EAT FOODS THAT ARE SIGNIFICANT SOURCES OF VITAMIN A.

3. ONLY 27% OF THE AMERICAN POPULATION REACH THE U.S. RDA FOR VITAMIN A THROUGH FOODS INGESTED.

4. ONLY 9% OF THE ADULT POPULATION REACH THE RECOMMENDED GUIDELINES FOR AT LEAST 5 VEGETABLE AND FRUIT SERVINGS PER DAY.

WITH THIS INFORMATION ALONE, IT IS CLEAR THAT THE NEED FOR VITAMIN SUPPLEMENTS IN THE AMERICAN DIET IS EXTREMELY GREAT.

VITAMIN SUPPLEMENTATION PLAN

Choose a palatable multi-vitamin that doesn't disturb your gastro-intestinal tract. Take one of these vitamins daily and add to it:

VITAMIN C
500 MG/DAY

THIS VITAMIN IS MOST IMPORTANT IN WOUND HEALING, THE IMMUNE SYSTEM, THE SKELETAL SYSTEM AND IT IS A POTENT ANTIOXIDANT.

BETA-CAROTENE
20,000 IU/DAY

LOWERS RISK OF LUNG CANCER AND CANCERS OF THE GI TRACT—ALSO ACTS AS AN ANTIOXIDANT.

VITAMIN B12
400 MCG/DAY

VITAMIN B12 IS IMPORTANT FOR REDUCING HOMOCYSTEINE, WHICH IS A PRODUCT IN THE BLOOD THAT IS VERY HARMFUL TO BLOOD VESSELS. WE WILL DISCUSS HOMOCYSTEINE LATER IN THIS BOOK.

VITAMIN B6
200 MG/DAY.

VITAMIN B6 ACTS AS ADJUNCT TO VITAMIN B12 AND FOLIC ACID IN PREVENTING HEART ATTACK AND STROKE; AND VERY IMPORTANT IN REDUCING HOMOCYSTEINE LEVELS.

FOLIC ACID
400 MCG/DAY

FOLIC ACID IS VERY IMPORTANT IN REDUCING HOMOCYSTEINE LEVELS AND DECREASING INCIDENCE OF HEART ATTACK AND STROKE; AND IMPORTANT IN REDUCING NEURAL TUBE BIRTH DEFECTS.

VITAMIN E
400 IU/DAY

REDUCES THE RISK OF CARDIOVASCULAR EVENTS I.E., HEART ATTACK AND STROKE—IMPORTANT IN HEALING ARTERIAL INTIMA WHICH IS THE LINING OF ARTERIES—REDUCES RISK OF CATARACTS, BOOSTS THE IMMUNE SYSTEM—HAS BEEN IMPLICATED IN DECREASING THE RISK OF CERTAIN TYPES OF CANCER.

SO, YOU SAY, "WOW, THAT IS A LOT OF PILLS TO TAKE EACH DAY." YES, BUT SINCE YOUR DAILY FOOD INTAKE IS SO VITAMIN POOR, IT IS IMPORTANT TO ADD THESE SUPPLEMENTS TO YOUR DIET TO MAINTAIN A HEALTHY BODY, PLUS YOU CAN REDUCE THE INCIDENCE OF HEART ATTACK AND STROKE BY AS MUCH AS 40%. WOULDN'T YOU RATHER TAKE SEVERAL VITAMINS EACH DAY THAN SUSTAIN A DAMAGING HEART ATTACK, STROKE, OR WORSE AND THEN TAKE SEVERAL PRESCRIPTION MEDICATIONS EACH DAY TO DEAL WITH YOUR DISEASE PROCESS?

It has been repeatedly shown through research studies that the antioxidant levels required to have a positive effect on protecting cells from the harmful effects of free radicals are significantly higher than the US RDA.

Vitamin E, a powerful antioxidant, in doses of 400 IU/day may reduce coronary disease by as much as 40%. This important information was reported in *The New England Journal of Medicine* by Harvard researchers involving 120,000 men and women. The current US RDA for Vitamin E per day is only 15 IU.

Thus, the need for vitamin supplementation is well established. However, one must not overindulge on vitamins because huge dosages of vitamins can, in some instances, cause harmful effects instead of beneficial results. The key word here is *moderation.* Apply it to everything you do: your exercise program, your new attitude, and certainly to your vitamin and mineral supplementation plan.

Recently, vitamin assays have become available via blood samples, which determine the level of certain vitamins present in your bloodstream. This information can be helpful to determine particular vitamin insufficiency states, but currently this test is quite expensive.

So, honor your commitment to health, observe the "Rule of Hand," continue your exercise program, and take your vitamin supplements each day. Another pill that can be very beneficial is an 81 mg enteric-coated aspirin taken daily, provided you are not allergic to aspirin. The aspirin acts as a blood platelet inhibitor, which in effect acts as a mild blood anticoagulant to allow the blood to be "slippery" and pass more easily over the rough spots on our arteries.

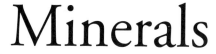

Minerals

From a nutritional standpoint, minerals are a major component to achieving and maintaining a state of wellness.

There are two categories of minerals, which have been determined to be important to your health. The minerals that are required in your daily diet in amounts greater than 100 mg/day are called Major minerals and minerals that are required in your diet less than 100 mg/day are termed Trace minerals.

All body tissues and internal fluids contain minerals of different varieties and varying quantities. Minerals are the main constituents of the bones and

teeth and are contained in the soft tissue, muscle, blood, nerves and brain cells as well.

Minerals are very important for many of the chemical and electrical reactions in the body,

MAJOR MINERALS ESSENTIAL FOR HUMAN WELLNESS
CALCIUM
PHOSPHOROUS
MAGNESIUM
SULFUR
SODIUM
POTASSIUM
CHLORIDE

and they play a significant role in the production of hormones and digestive secretions and the metabolism of food.

The best *natural* source of minerals is from the vegetables and fruits you eat. Plants are able to extract metallic minerals from the soil and assimilate these minerals into a water-soluble form, which our bodies can absorb and then utilize. However, as previously discussed, farming practices for the past 100 years have so depleted our soil of the minerals necessary for health that the harvested plants, fruits, and vegetables contain very little of the minerals we need.

This fact coupled with the known fact that the adult population eats insufficient amounts of fruits and vegetables daily, leaves the population in a chronic mineral insufficient state.

Thus, the obvious need for mineral supplements exists.

So how do you supplement your diet with the all-important minerals? Multi-mineral supplementation is available in pill form as well as in flavorful, easily digested liquid.

TRACE MINERALS: Trace minerals are the minerals that occur in amounts of less than 100 mg/day or in trace or tiny portions.

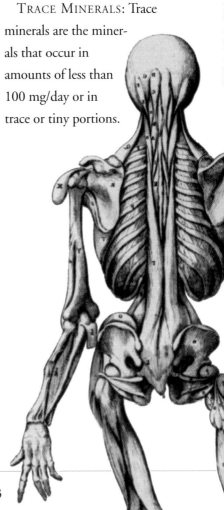

Their importance, however, is not to be minimized for they play major roles in health. Even tiny portions or a lack thereof can significantly affect your state of wellness. They are essential to the utilization of vitamins, and they act as catalysts in a variety of enzymatic reactions in essential body functions.

Most nutritional experts have identified 15 minerals that are necessary to maintain average health. However, there are another 85 minerals for which daily minimal requirements have not been established. It is quite possible that trace amounts of these 85 minerals may play a significant role in achieving the

TRACE ELEMENTS

These elements have been identified by nutritionists to play an integral role in human wellness.

MINERAL	ACTION	RDA/SAI*
BORON	BUILDING AND MAINTAINING BONE STRUCTURE	UNKNOWN
CHROMIUM	CONTROL BLOOD SUGAR	200 MG
COBALT	VITAMIN B 12 PRECURSOR	UNKNOWN
COPPER	RED BLOOD CELLS, ANTIOXIDANTS	3 MG
FLUORIDE	FIGHTS TOOTH DECAY, BUILDS STRONG BONES	4 MG
IODINE	THYROID FUNCTION	150 MG
IRON	HEMOGLOBIN IN RED BLOOD CELLS	15 MG
MANGANESE	ANTIOXIDANTS METABOLISM OF VITAMIN B 1 AND VITAMIN E PROTEIN DIGESTION	5 MG
MOLYBDENUM	GROWTH AND SKELETAL DEVELOPMENT	250 MCG
NICKEL	HORMONES, ENZYMES	UNKNOWN
SELENIUM	HEALTHY SKIN, ANTIOXIDANTS	70 MCG
ZINC	IMMUNE SYSTEM	15 MG

*RDA= RECOMMENDED DAILY ALLOWANCE / SAI = SAFE AND ADEQUATE INTAKE

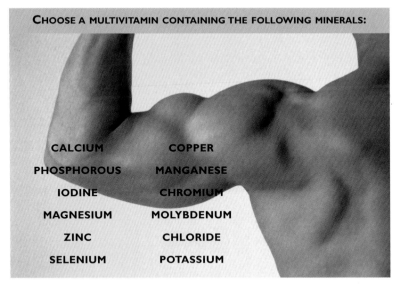

CHOOSE A MULTIVITAMIN CONTAINING THE FOLLOWING MINERALS:

CALCIUM	COPPER
PHOSPHOROUS	MANGANESE
IODINE	CHROMIUM
MAGNESIUM	MOLYBDENUM
ZINC	CHLORIDE
SELENIUM	POTASSIUM

best possible state of health.

Once again, due to dietary deficiencies in fruits and vegetables, not only are *vitamin supplements* necessary for your health and nutrition, but *mineral supplements* are equally as *vital.*

The best source of minerals are plant derived, for these minerals are water soluble and are easily digested and assimilated in your bodies. This type of mineral is called a hydrophilic mineral. For those of you who are averse to

"taking pills," there are certain liquid products available, which are most palatable and contain satisfactory amounts of vitamin and mineral supplements.

Do some checking, and use only those mineral products of hydrophilic derivation produced by reputable companies. And remember this is just a part of a healthy food design that *you* have decided to implement and that *you* are accountable for your health.

MAJOR MINERALS ESSENTIAL FOR HUMAN WELLNESS

CALCIUM

CALCIUM IS UTILIZED IN BUILDING AND MAINTAINING OUR SKELETAL STRUCTURE AND IS ESSENTIAL FOR HEALTHY BONES AND TEETH. IN ITS IONIZED FORM, IT IS IMPORTANT IN REGULATING ELECTRICAL IMPULSES IN YOUR HEART AND SKELETAL MUSCLES AS WELL AS AIDING IN LOWERING BLOOD PRESSURE AND ASSISTING IN THE NORMAL BLOOD CLOTTING MECHANISM. **IT IS NECESSARY TO PREVENT OSTEOPOROSIS.**

MAGNESIUM

MAGNESIUM IS VERY IMPORTANT IN THE ELECTRICAL ACTIVITY OF THE HEART AND IS NECESSARY FOR THE METABOLISM AND CORRECT UTILIZATION OF VITAMIN C AND CALCIUM. MAGNESIUM IS NECESSARY FOR THE COMPLEX CONVERSION OF SUGAR INTO ENERGY.

IRON

THE MAIN USE OF IRON IN YOUR BODY IS TO COMBINE WITH A SPECIFIC PROTEIN IN THE FORMATION OF HEMOGLOBIN, WHICH IS THE OXYGEN-CARRYING SYSTEM IN YOUR BLOOD AND IN THE FORMATION OF MYOGLOBIN, WHICH IS NECESSARY TO OXYGENATE THE MUSCLE CELLS.

IODINE

IODINE IS NECESSARY FOR THE DEVELOPMENT AND CONTINUED NORMAL FUNCTION OF THE THYROID GLAND, WHICH IS RESPONSIBLE FOR REGULATING THE BODY'S METABOLIC RATE.

COPPER

COPPER MUST BE PRESENT TO ABSORB AND UTILIZE IRON, AND IT IS AN IMPORTANT COMPONENT IN THE ELASTIC PROPERTIES OF YOUR TISSUES. IT IS NECESSARY FOR PROPER FORMATION AND MAINTENANCE OF BONE. COPPER ALSO IS VERY IMPORTANT IN THE OXIDATION PROCESS OF VITAMIN C WHICH IS ESSENTIAL TO THE HEALING PROPERTIES OF YOUR BODY.

ZINC

ZINC IS NECESSARY FOR BUILDING PROTEINS AND IT IS VITAL FOR THE DEVELOPMENT AND MAINTENANCE OF THE REPRODUCTIVE ORGANS. ZINC IS NECESSARY IN WOUND HEALING PROCESSES; IT AIDS IN THE NORMAL ELECTRICAL FUNCTION IN MUSCLE CONTRACTION, AND IT IS NECESSARY TO MAINTAIN NORMAL MENTAL ALERTNESS.

MANGANESE

MANGANESE PLAYS AN IMPORTANT ROLE IN ASSISTING THE ANTIOXIDANT AGENTS AND IS NECESSARY FOR METABOLISM OF VITAMIN B-1 AND VITAMIN E. MANGANESE IS UTILIZED IN THE BREAK DOWN OF AMINO ACIDS AND IS NECESSARY FOR PRODUCTION OF ENERGY IN THE METABOLISM OF FOOD STORES. IT ACTS AS A CATALYST IN THE BREAK DOWN OF FATS AND CHOLESTEROL, AND IT HELPS MAINTAIN SEX HORMONE PRODUCTION. MANGANESE IS NECESSARY FOR THE NOURISHMENT OF PERIPHERAL NERVES AS WELL AS THE CENTRAL BRAIN CELLS.

MAJOR MINERALS ESSENTIAL FOR HUMAN WELLNESS

CHROMIUM

CHROMIUM FUNCTIONS IN CONJUNCTION WITH INSULIN IN THE METABOLISM OF SUGAR AND IS IMPORTANT IN THE TRANSPORT MECHANISM OF AMINO ACIDS. IT AIDS THE ANTIOXIDANTS IN LOWERING CHOLESTEROL AND TRIGLYCERIDE LEVELS.

POTASSIUM

POTASSIUM FUNCTIONS WITH SODIUM IN A COMPLEX EXCHANGE IN THE KIDNEYS WHEREBY TOXIC BODY WASTE PRODUCTS ARE ELIMINATED. NORMAL LEVELS OF POTASSIUM ARE NECESSARY TO MAINTAIN PROPER ELECTRICAL IMPULSES THROUGHOUT THE BODY AND IT IS ESPECIALLY IMPORTANT IN MAINTAINING NORMAL HEART RHYTHM.

SELENIUM

SELENIUM IS IMPORTANT IN PRESERVING TISSUE ELASTICITY AND THROUGH ITS ANTIOXIDANT ASSISTANCE, SLOWS THE AGING AND HARDENING OF TISSUES. BY BEING AN ANTIOXIDANT NUTRIENT, SELENIUM HELPS PROTECT CELL MEMBRANES AND PREVENTS FREE RADICAL GENERATION, WHICH IS INJURIOUS TO BLOOD VESSELS. SELENIUM HAS BEEN REPORTED BY UNIVERSITY OF ARIZONA EPIDEMIOLOGIST, LARRY C. CLARK, TO POSSIBLY REDUCE THE RISK OF CANCERS OF THE PROSTATE, LUNG, AND COLON.

PHOSPHOROUS

PHOSPHOROUS IS INVOLVED IN THE MAINTENANCE OF THE ACID-BASE BALANCE OF THE BLOOD. IT PLAYS A MAJOR ROLE IN METABOLIZING CARBOHYDRATES, BUILDING PROTEINS, AND TRANSFERRING FATTY ACIDS AND FATS TO THE APPROPRIATE ORGANS AND TISSUES.

A WORD OF CAUTION is in order in taking minerals, per se, for the minerals may be in a form that is poorly digested and poorly absorbed and these are minerals from the soil which are usually in the metallic form.

THE BEST SOURCES OF MINERALS are PLANT DERIVED, because these minerals are water soluble and are easily digested and assimilated in your body. This type of mineral is called a hydrophilic mineral.

You should be aware, however, that even though many mineral supplements state there are over 70 minerals contained in the product, there frequently is no information relating to the source and type of minerals, so choose a supplement product of a reliable and reputable company.

Alcohol

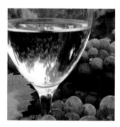

Alcohol should be consumed on a basis that is commensurate with the theme of this book— moderation.

Alcohol is the product of fermentation of a carbohydrate— an enzymatically controlled breakdown of carbohydrate into carbon dioxide and alcohol. If you choose to drink alcohol, it should be consumed on a basis that is commensurate with the theme of this book—*moderation.*

Be prudent in your assessment of moderation, and do not overindulge by not being truthful to yourself in regard to the amount of alcohol you consume.

Research indicates four ounces

of red wine two or three times per week may actually decrease your risk of stroke or heart attack. Other studies support similar findings. At the other end of the spectrum, however, studies have also shown that as few as seven drinks per week for women and 14 drinks per week for men can have a negative affect on health. If you have had alcohol-related problems in the past, you should avoid alcohol all together.

Daily overindulgence of

alcohol may lead to alcoholism or liver damage. Also, there is a higher incidence of cancer of the throat and the esophagus in chronic alcohol abusers. Excess alcohol inhibits the body's ability to absorb vitamins and in addition, promotes a muscle wasting process, particularly in older people.

Even though calorie counting is not an issue in this health design, alcohol carries a very high caloric value and if you are not careful in the amount of alcohol you consume, you may develop excess body fat storage even if the "Rule of Hand" is being carefully followed.

This thought is particularly important to those who consume large quantities of *beer.*

Consuming large quantities of alcohol over a period of time also precipitates other important mental and physical health risks in addition to those addressed above. So, keep a tight rein on your alcohol consumption and enjoy good health.

Exercise

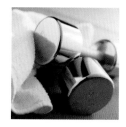

Do you want to look better, feel better, and have more energy and stamina at any age? Exercise!

Exercise is a key element for developing and maintaining healthy bodies at *all* ages. Exercise strengthens your body's musculature, which, of course, is the "engine" that drives your skeleton to motion upon an impulse from the nervous system.

Upon strengthening your musculature, you not only look better, but you feel better with more energy and stamina. Interestingly, a person with a lean body mass actually burns more calories at rest than an overweight/obese individual.

Also, many recent studies confirm that individuals, who exercise regularly exhibit increased brainpower and sharper mental activity. These findings were observed in people who had led sedentary lifestyles for many years and had become "fluffy" and overweight. Brain function was measured with sophisticated uptake studies in these sedentary people before initiating an exercise program,

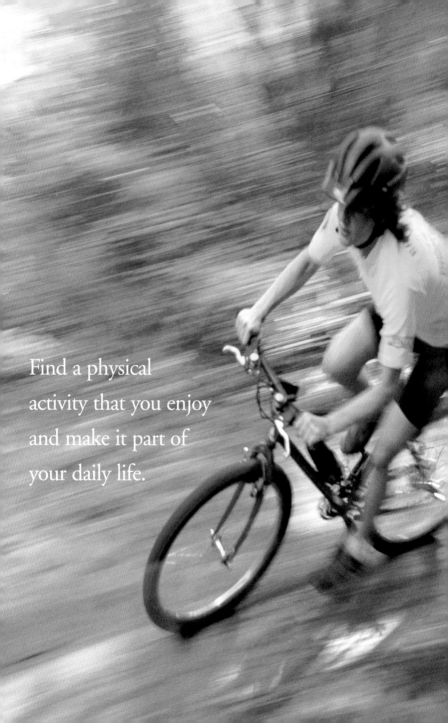

Find a physical
activity that you enjoy
and make it part of
your daily life.

then again at three months and at six months after starting the exercise program. In all of these individuals, a marked increase in brain activity and mental acuity occurred and some individuals showed as much as 30% increase in brain power.

Regular exercise is also beneficial in lowering your blood pressure. Many people have been able to have their high blood pressure medication discontinued after invoking and sustaining a regular exercise program.

Exercise will *naturally* dilate or open the arteries which lowers the resistance in blood vessels and this in turn, decreases the workload on the heart muscle. Thus, exercise in moderation may enhance your longevity, but it must be continued on a regular basis. Many people exercise less and less as they grow older. However, the older you get, the *more important* it is to exercise regularly.

I have already touched upon the improvement of brain function with regular exercise; but also, there may be some deterrent action against the development of

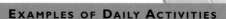

EXAMPLES OF DAILY ACTIVITIES

A LESS OPTIMAL EXERCISE PROGRAM, THAT DOES NOT CARRY THE BENEFITS OF AN ESTABLISHED, FORMAL EXERCISE PROGRAM, HAS BEEN OUTLINED BY THE US SURGEON GENERAL. SOME PEOPLE MAY FIND IT MORE ACCEPTABLE TO INCORPORATE THESE TYPES OF ACTIVITIES INTO THEIR LIFESTYLE.

WASHING AND WAXING A CAR	45-60 MINUTES
WASHING WINDOWS OR FLOORS	45-60 MINUTES
PLAYING VOLLEYBALL	45 MINUTES
GARDENING	30-45 MINUTES
WHEELING YOURSELF IN A WHEELCHAIR	30-40 MINUTES
WALKING 1-3/4 MILE	35 MINUTES
BASKETBALL (SHOOTING BASKETS)	30 MINUTES
BICYCLING	5 MILES IN 30 MINUTES
DANCING FAST (SOCIAL)	30 MINUTES
PUSHING A STROLLER	1-1/2 MILES IN 30 MINUTES
RAKING LEAVES	20 MINUTES
WALKING 2 MILES	30 MINUTES
WATER AEROBICS	30 MINUTES
SWIMMING LAPS	20 MINUTES
WHEELCHAIR BASKETBALL	20 MINUTES
BASKETBALL (PLAYING A GAME)	15-20 MINUTES
BICYCLING	4 MILES IN 15 MINUTES
STAIR WALKING	15 MINUTES

Alzheimer's Disease, which appears to develop more frequently, and earlier in the sedentary population.

Regular exercise not only strengthens the musculature, but it strengthens ligaments and joint structures, and it improves reaction time to accidents thus diminishing serious falls and injuries which plague the sedentary elderly population.

Who should exercise? *Everyone!*

This simply cannot be emphasized enough. It is extremely important for everyone to exercise at *some* level, even the severely physically limited. But before initiating any type of planned exercise program, see your physician for physical

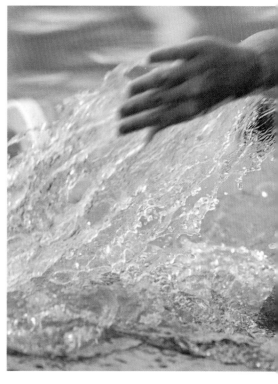

clearance. Also, you need to understand that if your most strenuous activity up until this time has been trotting to the refrigerator during a commercial, you will have to work your way into a healthy exercise routine. Your physician can help you accomplish this.

Remember—*start slowly.*

The best exercise programs are individually tailored by local hospital facilities, YMCAs,

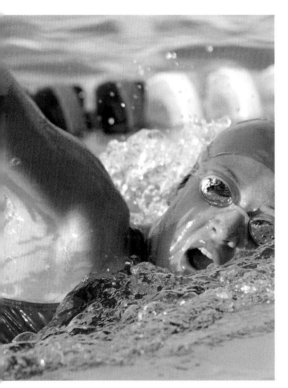

aquatic workouts for those who have severe joint problems.

So, there is really no reason to not exercise—just excuses.

Have a physical trainer outline a specific regimen for you and plan your days so that you may exercise vigorously for 20-30 minutes a minimum of four days per week. An important bit of advice is to choose an activity you enjoy. If you enjoy your workout, you are more apt to continue doing the activity and incorporate it into your daily

YWCAs, or private exercise facilities where certified physical trainers are employed. These programs generally have exercise facilities for all levels including

activities. This requires effort on your part and a *commitment.*

So, make this commitment and start today with a new attitude.

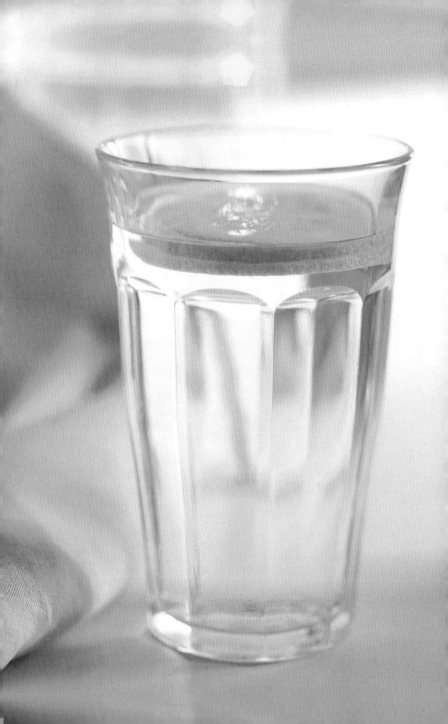

At the Movies

Drink water, not a soft drink. Water is good for your skin and better for your kidneys than any other liquid.

At the movies, almost invariably, when the overweight patron orders popcorn and drink from the concession stand, he or she will order a *huge tub* of *buttered popcorn* and *giant diet soft drink*. Apparently, the thought process here is something along these lines: "I can have a tub of buttered popcorn because I offset it with a diet drink." *Wrong!!*

This combination of massive carbohydrate and fat load completely upsets the insulin/glucagon mechanism and guess where this excess food energy goes? Directly through your *lips* to your *hips,* and there it is stored as excess body fat. The diet soft drink does not "offset" anything. It generally just adds more caffeine to your likely already over-caffeinated body.

Drink water, not a soft drink. Water is *good* for your *skin* and better for your kidneys than other liquids. Limit your intake of carbonated beverages the same as carbohydrate foods are limited. Drink soft drinks sparingly —regardless of whether the soft drink is "diet" or "regular."

Eating Out

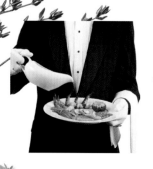

*When eating out, choose
your entrée with the protein
in mind first, eat slowly,
and drink plenty of water.*

Since eight out of 10 meals today are eaten outside the home, it is a key issue to monitor your portions and ratios of protein, carbohydrates, and fat when you are eating at a restaurant. This monitoring procedure is easily followed if you apply the information and principles previously discussed in this book.

Of course, you must arrive at the restaurant with a "wellness attitude" bolstered with commitment and accountability.

If you wish to have a glass of wine or cocktail before dinner, do so, *but one is enough.*

When the bread is served, you may have half a roll with a small amount of butter for flavor, but that means you have to give up your dessert. You must also offset the carbohydrate consumption by eating a lesser amount of carbohydrates with your entrée. Remember the "Rule of Hand."

You don't have to always be so rigid or controlled in your dietary habits. When ordering your meal, choose your entrée with the protein portion first in mind (meat, fish, chicken) then exchange the rice, pasta, or potatoes for steamed vegetables (carbohydrates). The cooking oils and salad dressing easily suffice for the necessary balancing fat portion. If the protein portion of your entrée is greater than allowed in the "Rule of Hand," take the residual portion home with you and consider incorporating it in tomorrow's breakfast, lunch, or dinner.

If you desire a dessert, feel free to indulge in whatever you like, but eat only a third to a half and

then share the remainder with your companions or simply discard what is remaining.

To *avoid over eating,* eat slowly and drink plenty of water. Try not to skip meals and avoid getting hungry by eating a balanced snack of 1/3 protein, 1/3 carbohydrate, 1/3 fat if you feel you *must* eat something between meals.

This design can and should be followed by everyone. *Just do it!*

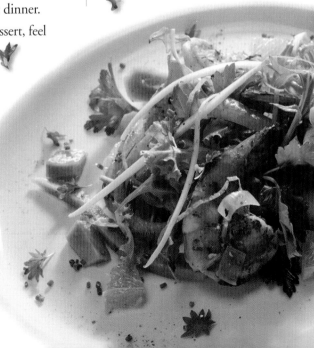

Homocysteine

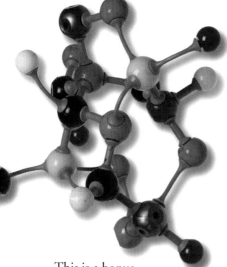

Contact your physician and insist that your serum homocysteine level be checked in addition to your lipid profile.

This is a bonus chapter for you and it could be the *most important* piece of literature you read in your lifetime.

Although the word "homocysteine" may not be familiar to you now, it is very likely that homocysteine will be named the culprit arterial destroyer and terminator of the future because its role is far more critical in the destruction of arteries than cholesterol.

Elevated levels of serum homocysteine result in injury to the arterial wall. Fatty substances (cholesterol) accumulate at that site, which is covered by circulating immune cells (monocytes) resulting in inflammation. At this point, arterial cells proliferate as part of the healing process, causing scarring or plaque formation. As further plaque formation occurs in the healing process, the arterial wall is narrowed, thus impeding blood flow resulting in the formation of blood clots or actual disruption (dissection) of the lining of the arterial wall. This results in an immediate obstruction of the artery, with potentially catastrophic results.

It is important to note that elevated serum homocysteine sets the stage for arterial wall injury and elevated serum cholesterol results in an abnormal and often times over zealous healing process (plaque formation).

Homocysteine is derived from the breakdown of methionine by your body. Methionine is an amino acid that abounds in animal protein and its use is to build and maintain body tissues.

During *normal metabolism,* any excess homocysteine is quickly recycled by liver conversion back into methionine or further metabolized for excretion

but *only* with the help of Vitamin B12, Vitamin B6 and folic acid.

Smoking and inactivity tend to raise homocysteine levels and certainly, a dietary deficiency of Vitamin B12, Vitamin B6, and folic acid results in often times rather significant elevations of serum homocysteine.

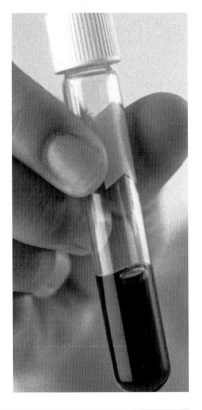

When heart disease runs in a family, the victims very often share a minor genetic flaw in the mechanism of homocysteine metabolism, but this flaw in most cases can easily be over-

subsequent investigations have clearly demonstrated that hyper-homocysteinemia (increased levels of homocysteine in the blood) is a strong and indepen-dent risk factor for atherosclero-

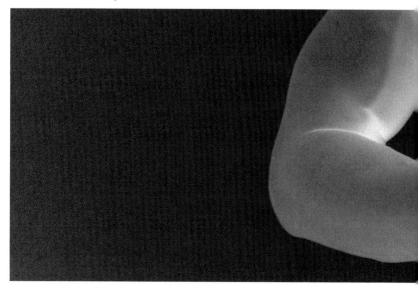

ridden by increased amounts of dietary Vitamin B12, Vitamin B6 and folic acid.

It was K. S. McCully who first made the clinical observation linking elevated plasma homo-cysteine concentrations with vascular disease, and many

sis and atherothrombosis.

Patients with mild elevations of serum homocysteine are typically asymptomatic until the third or fourth decades of life when pre-mature coronary artery or periph-eral vascular disease develops in addition to recurrent venous and

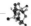

arterial thrombotic problems.

Vast numbers of epidemiological studies have confirmed and validated this relationship of hyperhomocysteinemia and vascular disease. For instance,

homocysteine level be checked in addition to your lipid profile. Remember, that *mild* elevations of homocysteine *are* hazardous, and that in the majority of incidences these elevations can be

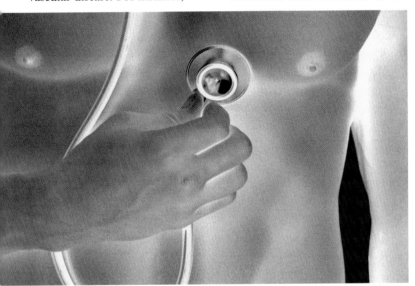

Clarke, et al. found the relative risk of coronary artery disease in patients with elevated serum homocysteine to be at least 24 times that in the control models.

Thus, my message to you is to contact your physician and request/insist that your serum

reversed with supplementation of Vitamin B12, Vitamin B6, and folic acid—a simple remedy.

Also remember that *you* are accountable for *you*, and your health is *your* responsibility. I hope I have driven this point home to you.

A Well Balanced You

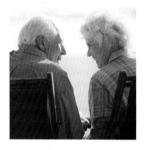

It is possible to nurture an inner strength that will help make you stronger and healthier than you ever realized you could be.

Throughout this book, we have focused on the importance of moderation in your diet and exercise plan. Moderation in the proteins, carbohydrates, and fats you eat, moderation in the amount of food you eat, moderation in the amount and type of exercise you do. *Moderation. Moderation. Moderation.*

Living a balanced life that nurtures your physical and mental health is a lifelong process that you can control. Other important areas you may wish to consider and further investigate for yourself include managing stress and getting in touch with your own spirtuality. It is possible to nurture an inner strength that will help make you stronger and healthier than you ever realized you could be.

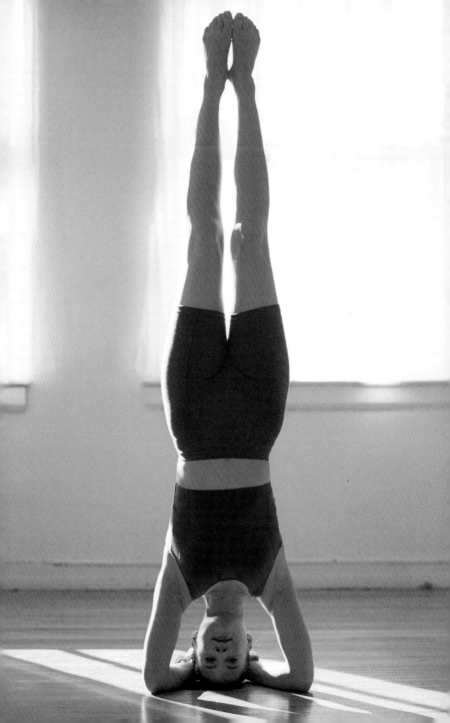

A LIST OF THINGS YOU CAN DO TO BUILD YOUR OWN HEALTH

EAT AND DRINK RIGHT

Follow the dietary recommendations in this book, focusing on the "Rule of Hand," and keeping the idea of balance and moderation in everything you do. Don't fall for "fad diets" that may cause you more harm than good.

DISCOVER YOUR OWN SPIRITUALITY

TAKE YOUR VITAMINS AND MINERALS

Be sure to give your body the important nutrients it needs to function at its optimum level, and supplement your diet with vitamins and minerals.

DEVELOP MEANINGFUL RELATIONSHIPS

Meaningful relationships connect us to ourselves, our families, our communities, and our world.

EXERCISE

Find an exercise plan that works for you and commit yourself to making that exercise routine a part of your daily life.

PUT TOGETHER A MEDICAL TEAM YOU TRUST

These professionals can help you identify and develop healthy habits that can help you live a healthier, longer life, and they can serve your health needs when you need them.

LEARN TO MANAGE STRESS

Avoid stress when you can and find your own way of relieving it.

PRACTICE MODERATION IN EVERY AREA OF YOUR LIFE

Summary

THE CARDIAC SURGEON'S
DIET & HEALTH DESIGN

This book has provided you with a sensible and workable health design which will help you achieve a healthy body weight, improved self-esteem, increased mental acuity, and the maximum state of wellness that is possible for you.

Proper eating habits require no weights and measurements other than the "Rule of Hand" as a guide for portions and ratios of protein, carbohydrates and fat. The proper allocation and portion of food is based primarily upon your size, which is best referenced by the size of your hand. You may think that the "Rule of Hand" is not enough food, but that is likely because you overeat! Employ the "Rule of Hand" and wait 10 minutes after you eat—you will not be hungry.

Attitude and commitment are the forerunners of this improved healthstyle. If you adopt a new attitude and follow the "Rule of Hand," exercise regularly, and take the correct vitamin and mineral supplements, you will notice a dramatic positive influence in many aspects of your life.

The End

References

Anderson R., Chromium and its role in lean body mass and weight reduction. *Nutr Rep. 1993: Vol.11: 41,46,48.*

Bendich A., Vitamin supplement safety issues. *Nutr Rep.1993: Vol.11:57,64.*

Bergsten P., Moura A., Atwater I., et al., Ascorbic acid and insulin secretion in pancreatic islets. *J Biol Chem. 1994: Vol. 269:1041-1045.*

Berr C., Nicole A., Godin J., et al., Selenium and oxygen-metabolizing enzymes in elderly community residents: A pilot epidemiologic study. *J Am Ger So. 1993: Vol. 41:143-148.*

Bland J., Antioxidants in nutritional medicine: Tocopherol, selenium and glutathione. *Yearbook of Nutritional Medicine. 1984-1985: New Canaan, CT. Keats Publishing Co., 213-237.*

Brattstrom L., Israelsson B., Norrving B, et al., Impaired homocysteine metabolism in early-onset cerebral and peripheral occlusive arterial disease: effects of pyridoxine and folic acid treatment. *Atherosclerosis. 1990: Vol. 81:51-60.*

Burke K., Skin cancer protection with L-selenomethionine. *Nutr Rep. 1992: Vol.10: 73, 80.*

Clarke R., Daly L., Robinson K, et al., Hyperhomocysteinemia: an independent risk factor for vascular disease. *N Engl J Med. 1991: Vol. 324: 1149-55.*

Dean R., Cheeseman K., Vitamin E protects against free radical damage in lipid environments. *Bioc Biop R 1987; 148:1277-1282.*

Den Heijer M., Koster T., Blom H.J., et al. Hyperhomocysteinemia as a risk factor for deep vein thrombosis. *N Engl J Med. 1996: Vol. 334:759-62.*

DIETARY GUIDELINES FOR HEALTHY AMERICAN ADULTS. *The American Heart Assoc'n. 1999.*

DIETARY INTAKE SOURCE DATA: UNITED STATES 1976-1980. *National Health Survey. March 1983: Washington, D.C. Series 11, No. 231. DHHS Publication no (PHS) 83-1681.*

Diplock A., Antioxidant nutrients and disease prevention: An overview. *Am J Clin N. 1991: Vol. 53: 189S-193S.*

Eagles J., Randall M. HANDBOOK OF NORMAL AND THERAPEUTIC NUTRITION. *1980: New York: Raven Press.*

Eastman C., Gullarte T., Vitamin B6, kynurenines, and central nervous system function: Developmental aspects. *J Nutr Bioc. 1992: Vol. 3: 618-631.*

England M., Gordon G., Salem M., *et al..* Magnesium administration and dysrhythmias after cardiac surgery. *J Am Med A. 1992: Vol. 268: 2395-2402.*

Garrison R. LYSINE, TRYPTOPHAN AND OTHER AMINO ACIDS. *1982: New Canaan,CT. Keats Publishing, Inc.*

Guilarte T,. Vitamin B6 and cognitive development: Recent research findings from human and animal studies. *Nutr Rev. 1993: Vol. 51:193-198.*

Handler S., Dietary fiber: Can it prevent certain colonic diseases? *Postgr Med.1983: Vol. 73: 301-307.*

Heaney R., Calcium in the prevention and treatment of osteoporosis. *J Intern Med. 1992: Vol. 231: 169-180.*

Heinrich, Elmer G. THE POWER OF PLANT DERIVED MINERALS. *1998.*

Kang S.S., Wong P.W., Malinow M.R, Hyperhomocysteinemia as a risk factor for occlusive vascular disease". *Ann Rev Nutr. 1992: Vol 12: 279-98.*

Kant A., Schatzkin A., Block G., et al., Food group intake patterns and associated nutrient profiles of the US population. *J Am Diet A. 1991: Vol. 91: 1532-1537.*

Keenan J., Wenz J., Ripsin C., et al., A clinical trial of oat bran and niacin in the treatment of hyperlipidemia. *J Fam Pract. 1992: Vol. 34: 313-319.*

Langford H., Sodium-potassium interaction in hypertension and hypertensive cardiovascular disease. *Hypertension 1991: Vol.17 (Suppl I): 21155-1157.*

Licata A., Jones-Gall D., Effect of supplemental calcium on serum and urinary calcium in osteoporosis patients. *J Am Col N. 1992: Vol. 11: 164-167.*

Lindenbaum J., Rosenberg I., Wilson P., et al., Prevalence of cobalamin deficiency in the Framingham elderly population. *Am J Clin N. 1994 Vol. 60: 2-11.*

Malinow M.R., Nieto F.J., Szkio M., Chambless L.F., Bond G., Carotid artery intimal-medial wall thickening and plasma homocysteine in asymptomatic adults: The atherosclerosis risk in communitics study. *1993: Vol. 87: 1107-13.*

Mantzoros C.S., The role of leptin in human obesity and disease: A review of current evidence. *Ann Intern Med. 1999: Vol. 130: 671-680.*

Matkovic V. and Ilich J., Calcium requirements for growth: Are current recommendations adequate? *Nutr Rev. 1993: Vol. 51: 171-180.*

McCarron D., Reusser M., The integrated effects of electrolytes on blood pressure. *Nutr Rep. 1991: Vol. 9: 57,62,64.*

McCully, K.S., Vascular pathology of homocysteinemia: implications for the pathogenesis of arteriosclerosis. *Am J. Pathol. 1969 Vol. 56: 111-28.*

McCully, K.S., Homocysteine and vascular disease. *Nat Med. 1996: Vol. 2: 386-9.*

Morris B., Blumshohn A., Mac Neil S., et al., The trace element chromium: A role in glucose homeostasis. *Am J Clin N. 1992: Vol. 55: 989-991.*

NATIONAL RESEARCH COUNCIL. RECOMMENDED DAILY ALLOWANCES. *1989: Washington, D.C. National Academy Press.*

Newhouse I., Clement D., Lai C., Effects of iron supplementation and discontinuation on serum copper, zinc, calcium and magnesium levels in women. *Med Sci Spt. 1993: Vol. 25: 562-571.*

Nygard O., Vollset S.E., Refsum H., et al., Total plasma homocysteine and cardiovascular risk profile: The Hordaland Homocysteine Study. *JAMA. 1995: Vol. 274:1526-1533.*

Nygard O., et al., Plasma homocysteine levels and mortality in patients with coronary artery disease. *N Engl J Med. 1997: 337:230.*

Oakley G.P. Jr, Erickson J.D., Adams M.J. Jr., Urgent need to increase folic acid consumption. *JAMA 1995: Vol. 274: 1717-8.*

O'Neill D., Barber R., Reversible dementia caused by vitamin B12 deficiency. *JAGS. 1993: Vol. 41: 192-199.*

Press R., Geller J., Evans G., The effect of chromium picolinate on serum cholesterol and apolipoprotein fractions in human subjects. *West J Med. 1990: Vol. 152:41-45.*

Rimm, Eric B., et al., Folate and Vit. B6 from diet and supplements in relation to risk of coronary heart disease among women. *JAMA. 1998: Vol. 279, No. 5.*

Saltzman E., Mason J.B., Jacques P.F., et al., B vitamin supplementation lowers homocysteine levels in heart disease. *Clin Res 1994: Vol. 42: 172A.*

Sandstead H., Zinc requirements, the recommended dietary allowance and the reference dose. *Sc J Work E. 1993: Vol. 19 (suppl 1): 128-131.*

Schectman G., Estimating ascorbic acid requirements for cigarette smokers. *Ann NY Acad. 1993: Vol. 686: 335-346.*

Sclhub J., Jacques P.F., Bostom A.G., et al., Association between plasma homocysteine concentrations and extracranial carotid-artery stenosis. *N Engl J Med. 1995: Vol. 332: 286-91.*

Selhub J., Jacques P.F., Wilson P.W., Rush D., Rosenberg I.H., Vitamin status and intake as primary determinants of homocysteinemia in an elderly population. *JAMA 1993: Vol. 270: 2693-2698.*

Shechter M., Kaplinsky E., Rabinowitz B., The rationale of magnesium supplementation in acute myocardial infarction. *Arch Int Med. 1992: Vol. 152: 2189-2195.*

Sies H., Stahl W., Sundquist A., Antioxidant functions of vitamins. Vitamins E and C, beta carotene, and other carotenoids. *Ann NY Acad 1992: Vol. 669: 7-20.*

Simon J., Vitamin C & Heart Disease. *Nutr Rep. 1992: Vol. 10: 57,64.*

Singh R., Rastogi S., Ghosh S., et al., Dietary and serum magnesium levels in patients with acute myocardial infarction, coronary artery disease and noncardiac diagnoses. *J Am Col N. 1994: Vol. 13: 139-143.*

Sowers M., Wallace R., Lemke J., The relationship of bone mass and fracture history to fluoride and calcium intake: A study of three communities. *Am J Clin N.* 1986: Vol. 44: 889-898.

Srikumar T., Johansson G., Ockerman P., et al., Trace element status in healthy subjects switching from a mixed to a lactovegetarian diet for 12 mo. *Am J Clin N.* 1992: Vol. 55: 885-890.

Stampfer M.J., Malinow M.R., Willett W.C., et al., A prospective study of plasma homocysteine and risk of myocardial infarction in US physicians. *JAMA.* 1992: Vol. 268: 877-81.

Stampfer M., Willett W., Homocysteine and marginal vitamin deficiency. *J Am Med A.* 1993: Vol. 270: 2726-2727.

Stampfer M.J., Malinow M.R., Can lowering homocysteine levels reduce cardiovascular risk? *N Engl J Med.* 1995: Vol. 332: 328-9.

Stevens J., Cai J., Juhaere, Thun M.J., Williamson D. F., Wood J.L., Consequences of the use of different measures of effect to determine the impact of age on the association between obesity and mortality. *AM J Epidemiol.* 1999: Vol. 150: 399-407.

Supplemental dietary potassium reduced the need for antihypertensive drug therapy. *Nutr Rev 1992: Vol. 50: 144-145.*

Toss G., Effect of calcium intake vs. other lifestyle factors on bone mass. *J Intern Med.* 1992: Vol. 231: 169-180.

Ueland P.M., Refsum H., Brattstrom L., "Plasma homocysteine and vascular disease. *Atherosclerotic Cardiovascular Disease, Hemostasis and Endothelial Function. 1992: New York, NY: Marcel Dekker Inc.:183-236.*

Ueland P.M., Refsum H., Plasma homocysteine, a risk factor for vascular disease: plasma levels in health, disease, and drug therapy. *J Lab Clin Med.* 1989: Vol. 114: 473-501.

Wabner C., Pak C., Modification by food of the calcium absorbability and physiochemical effects of calcium citrate. *J Am Col N.* 1992: Vol. 11: 548-552.

Wei Ming, Kampert J. B., Barlow Carolyn E., Nichaman M.Z., Gibbons, L. W., Paffenbarger R.S. Jr., Blair Steven N., Relationship between low cardiorespiratory fitness and mortality in normal weight, overweight, and obese men. *JAMA.* 1999: Vol. 282, No. 16.

Welch, George N. and Hoscalzo, Joseph., Homocysteine and atherothrombosis. *N Engl J Med. 1998: Vol. 338, No. 15.*

Winitz, M, Graff, J., Seedman, D.A., Effect of dietary carbohydrate on serum cholesterol levels. *Archives of Biochemistry and Biophysics. 1964: Vol. 108: 576-579.*

Yudkin, M.D. John C. , Ph.D., Professor of Nutrition, Queen Elizabeth College, London University.

Zinc and immunity. *Nutrition. 1994: Vol. 10: 79-80.*

ACKNOWLEDGEMENT

The publication of this book would not have been possible without the help and encouragement of my editor, Lorri Lagorin, designer, Karen Litchfield, and the staff of Creative Specialists, Inc. in Tulsa. CSI's projects have resulted in hundreds of new educational titles for health care professionals and consumers, year after year, since 1970.

Dr. B.P. Loughridge

PHOTO CREDITS:

ARTVILLE: 33, 44, 67

CORBIS: 48

EYEWIRE: III,V, 11, 18, 20, 21, 22, 23, 28, 29, 31, 48, 49, 59, 62, 63, 64, 74, 75

SCOTT MILLER, MILLER PHOTOGRAPHY: 26, BACK COVER

NATIONAL LIBRARY OF MEDICINE: 53

PHOTODISC: III, 7, 10, 12, 15, 18, 19, 24, 25, 30, 32, 34, 35, 38, 39, 41, 42, 46, 47, 50, 52, 57, 58, 60, 66, 68, 70, 71, 72, COVER, BACK COVER